The Lived Experience of Alternati

Mikel W. Hand

The Lived Experience of Alternative Graduate Nursing Education

A Qualitative Interpretive Phenomenological Study

VDM Verlag Dr. Müller

Impressum/Imprint (nur für Deutschland/ only for Germany)
Bibliografische Information der Deutschen Nationalbibliothek: Die Deutsche Nationalbibliothek verzeichnet diese Publikation in der Deutschen Nationalbibliografie; detaillierte bibliografische Daten sind im Internet über http://dnb.d-nb.de abrufbar.

Alle in diesem Buch genannten Marken und Produktnamen unterliegen warenzeichen-, marken- oder patentrechtlichem Schutz bzw. sind Warenzeichen oder eingetragene Warenzeichen der jeweiligen Inhaber. Die Wiedergabe von Marken, Produktnamen, Gebrauchsnamen, Handelsnamen, Warenbezeichnungen u.s.w. in diesem Werk berechtigt auch ohne besondere Kennzeichnung nicht zu der Annahme, dass solche Namen im Sinne der Warenzeichen- und Markenschutzgesetzgebung als frei zu betrachten wären und daher von jedermann benutzt werden dürften.

Coverbild: www.ingimage.com

Verlag: VDM Verlag Dr. Müller GmbH & Co. KG
Dudweiler Landstr. 99, 66123 Saarbrücken, Deutschland
Telefon +49 681 9100-698, Telefax +49 681 9100-988
Email: info@vdm-verlag.de
Zugl.: Malibu,Pepperdine,Diss.,2006

Herstellung in Deutschland:
Schaltungsdienst Lange o.H.G., Berlin
Books on Demand GmbH, Norderstedt
Reha GmbH, Saarbrücken
Amazon Distribution GmbH, Leipzig
ISBN: 978-3-8364-9840-1

Imprint (only for USA, GB)
Bibliographic information published by the Deutsche Nationalbibliothek: The Deutsche Nationalbibliothek lists this publication in the Deutsche Nationalbibliografie; detailed bibliographic data are available in the Internet at http://dnb.d-nb.de.

Any brand names and product names mentioned in this book are subject to trademark, brand or patent protection and are trademarks or registered trademarks of their respective holders. The use of brand names, product names, common names, trade names, product descriptions etc. even without a particular marking in this works is in no way to be construed to mean that such names may be regarded as unrestricted in respect of trademark and brand protection legislation and could thus be used by anyone.

Cover image: www.ingimage.com

Publisher: VDM Verlag Dr. Müller GmbH & Co. KG
Dudweiler Landstr. 99, 66123 Saarbrücken, Germany
Phone +49 681 9100-698, Fax +49 681 9100-988
Email: info@vdm-publishing.com

Printed in the U.S.A.
Printed in the U.K. by (see last page)
ISBN: 978-3-8364-9840-1

Table of Contents

LIST OF APPENDICES

Appendix A: Panel of Experts and Academic Qualifications

Appendix B: Sample Email Solicitation

Appendix C: Demographic Data Questionnaire

Appendix D: Lead in Question and Potential Probative Questions

Appendix E: Sample Composition

LIST OF TABLES

DEDICATION

I would like to dedicate this book to the loving memory of my two grandmothers Printhe Blackwell and Martha Hand. These two women taught me the value of faith, the power of prayer, and the importance of persistence. God called them to him during my undergraduate study, but he left their spirit with me. They guide me every single day of my life.

Grandma Hand I know that I am a better nursing faculty today because of your passion for teaching so many years ago. You taught me the value of being sure that not only information is conveyed, but also that learning takes place as a result. Grandma Blackwell I will never forget your words of encouragement or all the times you tucked me in after a long hard night shift. Both of you have left me a legacy for a lifetime.

ACKNOWLEDGEMENTS

There are many individuals that have been integral to the process of accomplishing this research. I would first like to acknowledge my esteemed chairperson Dr. Lois Blackmore. Dr Blackmore you are a visionary leader, risk taker, and a true friend. You were there when times were difficult and I simply wanted to give up. You helped to keep me focused throughout the course of the project and for that I am forever grateful.

I would also like to acknowledge my two outstanding committee members Dr. Randy Caine and Dr. Suzette Cardin. Dr. Caine I so much appreciate all of the support and wonderful suggestions that you have provided during the course of this research. You helped me to see light at the end of the tunnel when I could not see it alone. I am very proud to have you as a part of this committee and to have you as a friend. Your great accomplishments are a source of inspiration to me and make strive each day to be a better nursing faculty. Dr. Cardin I must say that when I first had you as a faculty at UCLA in 1998 I was not thinking that someday you would be on my doctoral committee, but I am so glad that you are. Your suggestion at the preliminary oral regarding the development of probative questions to be used in the interview was extremely beneficial and warded off disaster during the participant interview process. Thank you so much for volunteering to be a part of this research effort. You too are a powerful role model and a source of great inspiration.

Research participants do not pop out of the air, but rather professional assistance is often essential. I would like to thank Sandy Carter, Jean Pickus, Dr. Maryanne Garon, and Dr. Donna McNeese-Smith for assisting me in the process of soliciting participants for this study. I would not have been able to accomplish indirect solicitation without you. I know that each of my participants freely chose to participate in this study because they made a conscious decision to contact me after being given the information. Also, I want to thank Dr. McNeese-Smith for taking on the responsibility of Principal Investigator for one of the university sites. I will never forget all the emails we sent back and forth while you were in India, in order to complete the IRB paperwork. I could not have accomplished it successfully without you.

I would also like to acknowledge my life partner and very best friend Thomas Sheen. Tom you have no idea how important you support, love, and commitment have been to me in order for me to be able to complete doctoral study. You put up with me going through a masters program and then two years later returning to school for a doctorate. Your efforts go beyond the call of duty. I cannot promise this will be the last of my educational endeavors, but it will be for a while.

I would also be remiss not to acknowledge the wonderful work of Carla Bruce, Freelance Court Reporter. Carla your precision and accuracy in transcribing each of these interviews brought voice to the narrative and clarity to the meaning of the experience. You have no idea how invaluable your services have been in making this research possible.

Last but not least, I would like to acknowledge the entire faculty at Pepperdine University Graduate School of Education and Psychology who have contributed to my doctoral educational experience. Your wisdom and knowledge have made me a better person. I leave this program with a greater ability as an academician and a stronger feeling of the presence of God in my everyday life. To Christie Dailo our program administrator, you are God's angel planted here on earth. Thank you for what you do for each and every student. We could not do this without you.

Chapter 1: STATEMENT OF THE PROBLEM

Introduction, Background, and Significance

Recent trends in healthcare and an ever- increasing nursing shortage provide clear rationale for examining a broad array of issues related to comprehensive educational methodologies associated with professional nursing. Graduate nursing education at the master's level is no exception. Master of Science in Nursing programs prepare nurse educators, clinical nurse specialists, nurse practitioners, nurse anesthetists, nurse midwives, and administrators. Each of these challenging roles requires educational preparation beyond the baccalaureate level. This has not always been the case throughout history, but changes in regards to national certification requirements and state board regulations have caused this transition to occur.

There are numerous options from which an applicant may choose in order to attend a Master of Science in Nursing (MSN) program. These include a traditional full time day program, part time day or evening options, and alternative educational programs. Alternative programs employ a variety of instructional strategies including an intense accelerated curriculum, team learning, online classrooms and discussion groups, and others.

After careful consideration of the available educational options, many students choose to pursue degrees in alternative MSN programs. These programs present an array of benefits and challenges, which differ from traditional programs.

Statement of the Problem

Alternative MSN programs have been accepted as the academic norm and as such are worthy of in depth examination (Ali, Hodson-Carlton, & Ryan 2004). Life circumstances, which cause students to select these over traditional programs and the factors they deem critical to their academic success, should be of concern to nursing programs of every variety. According to the

American Association of Colleges of Nursing White Paper (2003), there will be more than one

million vacant positions for registered nurses in the United States by 2010. Of these, 39% are

positions requiring a baccalaureate or higher degree.

The issue of an aging workforce is also present in nursing academia. An aging faculty

workforce has compounded this problem by increasing the vacancy rate as a result of retirement.

According to the *White Paper (2003),* the national mean age of nursing faculty steadily increased

over ten years (1993 to 2003) from 49.7 to 53.3 years of age for doctorally prepared and from 46

to 48.8 years of age for masters. The significance of these findings rests in the ability to educate

nursing students with a sufficient number of academically qualified faculty. Faculty shortages

serve as a stimulus for colleges and universities to consider alternative ways of educating

students in order to make the most appropriate use of available resources and to contribute to the

future pool of academically qualified nursing faculty.

Alternative programs for nursing education are not an isolated concept. A 2002 survey of

162 nursing programs conducted by the National League of Nursing Accrediting Commission

indicated that the majority of the respondents were either engaged in alternative methods of

instruction or had plans in to do so in the future (Ali et al., 2004).

Existing literature related to alternative MSN programs focuses on specific issues such as

measurable outcomes, convenience, and accessibility. Limited attention is given to the individual

student's experience or life circumstances that precipitated their choosing an alternative

presentation of the curriculum Mueller (2001) stated:

There is a growing demand for masters prepared nurses to meet the health care needs of

the population. However, adult students find that multiple role responsibilities make it difficult to participate in the leisurely pace of the youth centered model of traditional

higher education. (p. 1)

With this in mind, there is a need to both describe the phenomenon of the student learning

experience in an alternative MSN program and understand the essence of meaning associated

with this lived experience and its' impact on the student. According to Felder and Brent (2005):

Students have different levels of motivation, different attitudes about teaching and

learning, and different responses to specific classroom and instructional practices.

The more thoroughly instructors understand the differences, the better chance they have

of meeting the diverse needs of all their students. (p. 57)

Lived experiences of student learning differ for each individual student and gaining insight into

these experiences is essential in addressing the individual needs of a diverse student population.

Purpose of the Study

The purpose of the study was to explore through formal inquiry the phenomenon of the

student learning experience in an alternative Master of Science in Nursing Program in order to

gain an understanding of the essence of meaning associated with this lived experience and its

impact on the student. For the purpose of this study the term alternative refers to programs that

employ methods of instruction such as online education, team learning, and/or accelerated

curriculum (Kozlowski, 2002). In the same context, student learning experience refers to the

entirety of that experience with inclusion of life circumstances that have influenced the student's

selection of the particular alternative program and the factors that they deemed critical to

academic success.

6

Method

The design for this study was based on similar research conducted by Mueller (2001). Mueller's research examined the phenomenon of the student learning experience in an online graduate nursing course. The participants in Mueller's study were students who were either currently enrolled in an online graduate nursing course or had previously taken course in the past year at one mid-western university (Mueller, 2001). This study expanded the examination of the phenomenon of the student learning experience by examining a sample of participants who had recently (within the last 3 years) completed their graduate degree program and included representation from three different university programs.

A qualitative interpretive phenomenological approach was utilized. Phenomenology examines the essence of a specific life experience and seeks to find the meaning of that experience (Polit, Beck, & Hungler, 2001). The researcher actions and the ultimate goal in this methodology were appropriate to answer the research questions in the study. The research methodology will be described in detail in chapter 3.

Research Questions

In order to comprehensively explore the lived student learning experience in an alternative MSN program, four major areas will be examined. Four main research questions guided the research in this study. They were as follows:

1. What were the five primary life circumstances that influenced the decision to select an alternative MSN program over that of a traditional program?

2. What were the three major underlying themes or elements in an alternative MSN program that students deemed critical to their success?

7

3. Which four primary underlying themes facilitate a description of the overall student learning experience in an alternative MSN program?

4. What are the four primary underlying themes that facilitate a description of why the student did not select a traditional MSN program?

Each of the questioned contains numeric parameters within them not for the purpose of forcing the data to fit into a specified mold, but rather to assist the researcher in framing those themes that provide the most textured description and data source. In order to answer these research questions, it was essential to provide a comprehensive explanation and definition of integral terminology prior to data collection.

Definition of Terms

The concepts and definitions essential to this study will be discussed in this section. The first concept of interest is that of life of life circumstances. *Life circumstances* are specific conditions such as family and parenting responsibilities, job requirements, geographical constraints and other elements that a graduate student might consider in the selection of a particular graduate program. These factors may influence the choice of an alternative MSN program.

Interpretive phenomenology is defined as a research tradition that uses "the lived experiences of individuals as a tool for better understanding the social, cultural, political, and historical context in which these experiences occur (Polit et al., 2001).

The term *Alternative MSN program* will refer to a graduate nursing program that employs methods of instruction such as accelerated course schedules, web based instruction, and especially off-site, on-line electronic instructional methods and materials (Kozlowski, 2002). In the past these methodologies have been alternative forms of instruction, but in the last decade they have been embraced as normal curriculum alternatives. Curriculum alternative can affect the learning experiences of the students.

Bracketing refers to the process of identifying and setting aside preconceived beliefs, and assumptions in order to view data in pure form (Polit et al., 2001). The practice of bracketing was not used as part of this study as it is impossible to suspend ones existence in the world and the attempt to bracket prior assumptions places the researcher in the position in not being open to the meaning of the experience of the participants.

Content validity within this study refers to the list of potential probative questions, demographic questionnaire and the extent to which they evaluate they all of the major elements of the phenomenon under examination (Burns & Grove, 2003). Content validity of both the potential probative questions and the demographic questionnaire were established by an expert panel consisting of five doctorally prepared nurse educators (Appendix A).

External validity within this study refers to the extent to which "findings from an investigation can be applied to other situations" (Merriam, 1993, p. 5). Within the realm of qualitative research, the individuals in those situations determine external validity. It would be unreasonable for the researcher to speculate how the findings obtained in this study would apply to other settings.

The *overall Student learning experience* is the phenomenon of the social learning experience in which the student engages in learning (Merriam & Caffarella, 1999). This phenomenon is an examination of the entirety of the alternative MSN experience. The learning experience of a student in a traditional classroom might differ from those taking an online course in terms of the amount and type of faculty/student interaction, learning activities, and instructional materials.

9

An *online course* is an instructional modality that takes place in a virtual classroom accessible by means of the Internet and university required software (George, 2002). This type of course may or may not involve face-to-face interaction. There is also a different variation of the online course. This variation is a hybrid modality. The *hybrid modality* refers to a course of instruction that involves both face to interaction and online work in a virtual classroom (Lorenzo, 2003). Communication in a virtual classroom might be either synchronous or asynchronous.

Synchronous communication is communication that occurs between students and faculty at the same time via the internet (Kozlowski, 2002). *Asynchronous communication* is electronic communication that involves delayed interaction between and among the participants in the classroom (Kozlowski, 2002). Examples of delayed interaction include newsgroup postings, message boards, and threaded discussion.

Reliability within this study refers to the degree to which the findings and conclusions derived from the study are consistent with the data collected (Merriam, 1993).

Triangulation within this study refers to the use of two or more data sources in order to establish validity and reliability (Burns & Grove, 2003). Stake (2003) further clarifies the process of triangulation as a process of using individual perceptions of a phenomenon to clarify meaning and different ways in which the phenomenon is being seen. In this study, participants were selected from three MSN programs, each at different universities in order to incorporate triangulation. Each of the programs is very different and as such the lived experience of the student differs.

Web casting refers to "a new educational technology used to deliver audio and video presentations via the Internet. It enables learners to participate in a live class via personal computers" (DiMaria-Ghalili, Ostrow, & Rodney, 2005, p. 11).

This section has provided the basic definitions involved in the phenomena integral to students who choose an alternative MSN program. The most appropriate methodological design to use to study the students experience is interpretive phenomenology.

Limitations of the Study

This study was limited to the three university programs from which the participants were selected and only included participants who had graduated from the specific MSN program tracks that utilized alternative methods of instruction as defined in this study. In addition, this study only examined the phenomenon of the lived student learning experience in the context in which it is shared by the participants. External validity of the conclusions derived from this study can only be determined by the consumer of the research, as it is unreasonable for the researcher to attempt to determine how these conclusions would apply in other situations or settings (Merriam, 1993). Fraenkel and Wallen (2001) stated "it is the practitioner, rather than the researcher, who judges the applicability of the researcher's findings and conclusions, who determines whether the researcher's findings fit his or her situation" (p. 447).

One additional area of limitation for this study was an academic requirement resulting in the inability of the researcher to gain independent understanding of the phenomenon of lived experience of student learning prior to exhaustive literature review. Van Manen (1990) provided clarification as to the rationale for this limitation.

> The question is whether one should turn to such phenomenological human science sources in the initial or in the later phases of one's research study. If one examines existing human science sources at the very outset then it may be more difficult to suspend one's interpretive understanding of the phenomenon. It is sound practice to attempt to address the phenomenological meaning of a phenomenon on one's own first. (p. 76)

Assumptions

These assumptions served as the basis for this study and are congruent with the interpretive phenomenological research methodology. These assumptions were not be suspended or set aside by bracketing (Polit et al., 2001), but were considered as integral to the process of interpreting and understanding the phenomenon. Heidegger (1962) stated:

Consequently, if we inquire about Being-in as our theme, we cannot indeed consent to nullify the primordial character of this phenomenon by deriving it from others—that is to say, by an inappropriate analysis, in the sense of a dissolving or breaking up. (P.170)

Van Manen (1990) stated "it is better to make explicit our understandings, beliefs, biases, assumptions, and theories" (p. 47). The purpose of making these assumptions explicit is to come to terms with them rather than suspending or holding them at bay.

These assumptions included the following:

1. The researcher has prior life experiences, ideas, and experiences related to the phenomenon. These will influence the researcher's interpretation of the data and serve to contribute to the essence of meaning.

2. All participants will be valued equally concerning the truths revealed in the narrative interviews conducted as a part of this study (Mueller, 2001).

3. Individuals' realities are influenced by the world in which they live (Lopez & Willis, 2004).

4. Individuals are constantly faced with choices even though the outcomes of the choices are often unclear (Solomon, 1987).

5. Human beings are capable of self- determination and interpretation.

Summary

Chapter 1 has presented an introduction, background of the study, statement of the problem, purpose, research questions, and a limited description of the research procedures. In addition, key assumptions serving as the basis for the study were also presented. Chapter two will present a review of the literature focusing on historical perspectives of alterative education and the virtual campus, key characteristics of adult learners, and program delivery methods. Chapter Three will detail the research methodology to be used in this study. Chapter four will present the analysis of the research study and key findings derived from the data. Chapter Five will identify and summarize implications and directions for further research.

Chapter 2: REVIEW OF THE LITERATURE

Introduction

Consistent with university requirements, chapter two will present a comprehensive review of the literature. When considering critical components to include in this literature review, it is important not only to address specific literature related to alternative education, but to also consider sources that address the philosophical and methodological concerns associated with interpretive phenomenology

The areas of focus for the literature review include lived experience and phenomenology, the interpretive phenomenological research approach, historical perspectives of alternative education and the virtual campus, program delivery methods, and key characteristics of adult learners.

Interpretive Phenomenology

Philosophical Orientation

It is important to remember that phenomenology is not only a research method, but also a philosophy. "Phenomenologists view the persons as integral with the environment. The world is shaped by the self and also shapes the self" (Burns & Grove, 1997, p. 71).

Interpretive phenomenology adheres to a constructivist interpretivist philosophical paradigm (Mueller, 2001):

Both the researcher and the participants bring their values and beliefs to the experience. Additionally the research experience is in itself another created context of interaction between researcher and participants. Scientific knowledge is always a situated perspective that is created as it occurs and therefore is unique and context bound. People create (construct) their own realities. The interpretivist paradigm adds assessment of the meanings to the traditional observation of human behavior (p. 24).

Within the constructivist view, reality is unique to each individual because it is created as it occurs (Denzin & Lincoln, 1994). Human beings create their reality and both the researcher and the participant bring their beliefs, assumptions, and values to the interaction. As a result, two people never experience the same situation in exactly the same way.

"Methodologically the constructivist paradigm adopts a hermeneutic and dialectic approach (Appleton & King, 1997, p. 15). Its' focus extends beyond merely the aspect of description to a level of understanding the core meaning of the constructions. There is a clear recognition within constructivism that others may hold beliefs that are different from the researcher.

Polit et al., (2001) noted that phenomenology has its base in a philosophical tradition developed by Husserl & Heidegger. This approach emphasizes examining life experiences and identifying the essence of them. Husserl (as cited in Giorgi, 1985) states that the guiding theme of phenomenology is "to back to the things themselves" (p. 8).

Schools of Phenomenology

Polit et al., (2001) discussed two schools of phenomenology, descriptive and interpretive. Each school is based on a primal question. Descriptive phenomenology primarily emphasizes the question: What do we know as persons? This question focuses on the meaning of the experience. Interpretive phenomenology moves beyond the realm of descriptive phenomenology and seeks to answer the question: what is being? It seeks to interpret and understand, rather than merely describe the experience.

15

McMillan and Schumacher (2001) stated, "phenomenological studies of a lived experience emphasize textual descriptions of what happened and how a phenomenon was experienced" (p. 490). The research report from this type of study will describe the experience of each participant, including the researcher. The essence of the experience is captured as a statement of meaning, describing the common experience.

Phenomenological Data Collection and Analysis

Burns and Grove (1997) suggested that data in a phenomenological study is collected through various approaches including researcher observations, interviews, videotaped observation, and written descriptions of the phenomenon provided by participants. Each approach lends an additional opportunity to gain additional understanding and aid in the interpretation of the phenomenon.

Interpretive phenomenology incorporates the use of hermeneutics. The word hermeneutics is a derivative of the word Hermes, a Greek god who was responsible for interpreting messages between gods (Lopez & Willis, 2004). During the reformation, hermeneutics were used in biblical criticism. This method has been further expanded in the social sciences for the purpose of gaining greater understanding of context and meaning of a particular phenomenon (Hoy, 1985). According to Hogan (nod.),

A hermeneutically disciplined understanding on this account would educate the learner-as interpreter in two ways-by disclosing in each instance something new about what the interpreter is attempting to understand and also something new about the learner himself/herself. Previously undetected biases, as well as new insights, might thus be progressively disclosed about the learner and what addresses the learner's efforts. These disclosures might be surprising, or disquieting, or satisfying or inspiring, or otherwise

challenging for learners.

(par. 5).

According to Lopez and Willis (2004), "hermeneutics goes beyond description of core concepts

and looks for essences of meaning in common life practices" (p. 728).

Creswell (1998) identified seven key steps in a phenomenological study as follows:

- Introduction (problem, questions)
- Research procedures (a phenomenology and philosophical assumptions, data collection, analysis, outcomes, analysis)
- Significant statements
- Meanings of statements
- Themes of meanings
- Exhaustive description of phenomenon (p. 67).

Polit et al., (2001) identified seven key steps in the analysis of data within an interpretive

phenomenological study:

1. Reading all of the interviews or texts for an overall understanding.
2. Preparation of interpretive summaries of each interview.
3. Analysis of selected transcribed interviews or texts by a team of researchers.
4. Resolution of any disagreements on interpretation by going back to the text.
5. Identification of common meaning by comparing and contrasting the texts shared practices.
6. Emergence of relationships among themes.
7. Presentation of a draft of the themes, along with exemplars for the text to the team; responses and suggestions are incorporated into the final draft. (p. 393- 394)

Cohen et al. (2000) brought further clarity to the process of data analysis by articulating

that data analysis begins during the process of the interview as the researcher is considering what

is being said, considering meanings, and developing preliminary labels for those meanings. The

process then moves to immersion as the researcher reads through the data several times. The

researcher then begins the process of data transformation or reduction. During this time, decisions are made concerning what is and is not pertinent as well as how data should be grouped concerning the specific topic. Data is then examined line by line and tentative theme labels are placed in the margins of the text. The next phase of the process involves writing and rewriting transforming a comparison of the themes to a coherent picture of the essence of meaning of the experience.

Lived Experience and Phenomenology

Phenomenology is the study of lived experience (Van Manen, 1990). It focuses on gaining a greater understanding of the meaning over daily life experiences.

Phenomenology asks, "What was this or that kind of experience like?" It differs from almost every other science in that it attempts to gain insightful descriptions of the way we experience the world pre-reflectively, without taxonomizing, classifying, or abstracting it. So phenomenology does not offer us the effective possibility of effective theory with which we can now explain and or control the world, but rather it offers us the possibility of plausible insights that bring us in more direct contact with the world (Van Manen, 1990, p. 9).

Van Manen (1990) provides six concrete suggestions to the researcher in attempting to produce a plausible description of lived experience:

1. You need to describe the experience as you lived through it. Avoid as much as possible explanations, generalizations, or abstract interpretations. For example it does not help to state what caused your illness, why you like swimming so much, or why you feel that children tend to like to play outdoors more than indoors.
2. Describe the experience from the inside, as it were; almost like a state of mind: the feelings, the mood, the emotions, etc.
3. Focus on a particular example or incident of the object of experience: describe specific events, an adventure, a happening, a particular experience.
4. Try to focus on an example of the experience which stands out for its vividness, or as it was the first time.

18

5. Attend to how the body feels, how things smell (ed), how they sound (ed) etc.
6. Avoid trying to beautify your account with fancy phrases or flowery terminology (p. 64-65).

Van Manen (1990) noted that any lived experience may be used to uncover a thematic description of the phenomenon to which they are related, but obviously some descriptions will be a richer source of information than others. In attempting to obtain the richest description of the lived experience the researcher may exercise conscious selection of certain "subjects, elements, or events to include in the study" (Burns & Grove, 2003, p.253).

Historical Perspectives, the Virtual Campus, and Generational Differences

Alternative education is not a new concept and has existed for hundreds of years. According to Higher Education (2002):

Although to many, distance education may seem a new phenomenon, various earlier forms began in the late 1800s and has been a part of many institutions s since the 1900s, as has the tradition of faculty traveling to off campus locations to meet local students. (p. 1)

Bates and Poole (2003) noted that alternative education has been around for centuries "For Christians St. Paul's Epistles to the Corinthians and the Romans in the first century could be considered a form of distance education. In 1840 Isaac Pittman started to use the Penny Post to teach the Phonographic shorthand he invented." (p. 94)

Bronson and Harriman (2000) noted that the first correspondence course offered by the University of Wisconsin in 1891 was by means of the pony express. This early effort has drastically evolved into what is now known as distance education. New technological developments have expanded upon this rudimentary concept.

19

The invention and evolution of computer technology has taken alternative education to a higher level of sophistication. One of these advances is the development of the concept of a *virtual campus*. The "virtual campus" is defined by Brogdon (2002) as a "centralized online learning space with administrative, pedagogical, and service functions. Its' purpose is to provide an integrated learning environment that responds to the unique and varied needs of a distant, mobile, and geographically diverse learning community" (p. 24). The virtual campus may also be identified as a metaphor for the electronic, teaching, learning, and research environment created by utilizing a variety of technologies including the Internet, computer mediated communication, multimedia, groupware, video on demand, and other technologies (Kay, 1995).

Alternative masters degree programs that utilize online instruction as one of their modalities incorporate two methods of interaction. These are synchronous and asynchronous communication. According to Kozlowski (2002),

> Synchronous learning is also termed real time learning. During scheduled activities, the student and teacher are in different geographical locations and are linked by some form of audio and or video communication system. With synchronous learning technology it is possible for the main classroom to be in Chicago, while offsite classrooms are scattered throughout the state, region, country and even internationally. (p. 42)

In contrast, asynchronous interaction between students and faculty does not take place simultaneously, but rather by means of electronic mail, bulletin boards, online list servers, and electronic newsgroups. George (2002) noted that a typical alternative degree program might employ one or both of these types of interactions.

Alternative methods of instruction have progressed far beyond correspondence courses delivered via the Pony Express. Bogie and Guilbert (2005) presented a unique approach taken by one Australian university. Every degree-seeking student, regardless of his or her major must take one fully online course as part of his or her degree program. In addition, every course taught at this university has some aspect of content presented in the online format.

Jeffries (2005) brought attention to the current direction of technology in nursing education:

The incorporation of new technology, alone or in combination with other methods reflects the direction of nursing education. Different types of technology are being used in today's classrooms laboratories, and or clinical sites to promote more realism in the practice environment, enhance the learning outcomes, and promote safe patient care environments in clinical practice. To keep up with our changing society and the technological advances in nursing practice, nurse educators will have to be creative in developing new, innovative models of teaching. Nurse educators will also need to be mindful of educational research, as these new methods are incorporated into the teaching-learning process

Just as nursing practice has changed dramatically during the past decade, so has the approach to nursing education. Educators needs to make certain they are informed about the possibilities of new technology, its' usefulness in enhancing student education, and the progress of educational research efforts conducted to guide new models of nursing education. (p.3)

In the process of examining historical perspectives, generational differences of students are worthy of consideration in relationship to the amount and type of interaction and feedback that students expect in a learning experience. Wagschal (1997) identifies generation X as individuals born between 1961 and 1981. Costello, Lenholt, and Stryker (2004) indicated that although characterized as highly independent, the generation X age group typically had a high demand for feedback and faculty interaction, as well as the expectation of a personalized educational experience. In addition, this age group has limited interest in the theoretical aspect of education and a stronger focus on concise practical information with a concise application.

Johnson and Romenello (2005) expanded the exploration of generational differences to include "Millenials (Born 1982-2002)" (p. 215). This group of individuals differs from generation X in that they have grown up with computer technology, electronic libraries, and has familiarity with team learning. In addition, this generation has a demand for immediacy in relationship to instructional feedback.

Program Delivery Methods

Alternative educational programs vary greatly in the methods of delivery. In order to perform a broad examination of delivery methods, an interdisciplinary multi-educational level examination will be presented. This examination included not only delivery methods used in nursing academia, but also those used in occupational therapy and education.

Wambach et al. (1999) described the delivery method at the University of Kansas School of Nursing utilized to provide a graduate level primary care nurse practitioner program via an online modality. Each course in the program is web based and has a uniform resource locator (URL). After the student locates the homepage, there are a variety of links to reach the course syllabus, objectives, videotaped lectures, assigned learning activity, and course related websites. All coursework is equivalent in content to the on campus program and is completed within a normal sixteen-week semester. Students are free to do their assignments at any time as long as they meet the assignment deadlines, as well as other course requirements.

Levin, Levin, Buell, and Waddoups, (2002) presented the delivery method used by the Master of Education program at the University of Illinois in Champagne-Urbana. This program utilizes a combination of both asynchronous and synchronous methods of interaction. Course descriptions, syllabi, and expectations are posted on a website. Instructors utilize the Web Board conferencing system for asynchronous discussions and text chat sessions. Electronic mail is utilized for one on one correspondence. Video taped lectures are streamed via an online video replay program Real Player. All of these methods are not utilized for the educational experience of the student, but to demonstrate use of education technology in practice.

Zlotolow (2002) described the program delivery method used by the Masters in Occupational Therapy program at San Jose State University. This 2-year program begins with an on campus orientation for the purpose of introduction to technology being used in the program and relationship building within the student cohort. All of the coursework is completed entirely online. The students come to the campus at the end of the 1st year for a 3-day workshop. The purpose of this workshop is to build the community of the online cohort. This time provides faculty and students the opportunity to strengthen existing online relationships.

Lorenzo (2003) points out that many programs incorporate a hybrid structure such as that used in the nursing program at Massachusetts Bay College. This program utilizes the Blackboard software for lectures and discussions, and a website for course syllabi and lecture notes. In person interaction with faculty takes place for the purpose of giving examinations and for clinical laboratory experience. The purpose of clinical laboratory experience is for the student to practice hands on patient care skills, which are less effectively evaluated by means of an online method.

Sykes (2003) described the synchronous delivery method used by the Doctor of Philosophy in Nursing, Cancer Research Program at the University of Utah. Students attend class from their home or preferred location twice weekly. Students are able to see their professor and classmates, as well as interact in real time. The goal of this program is the same as that of the program delivered by the university "to provide students with skills necessary to conduct scientific research and help improve patient care" (p.3).

Carter (2003) presented a blended approach to distance education used by one Canadian university:

Most classes are print based, interaction between the instructor and the students regularly occur via different electronic means including course specific listservs, and regular telephone contact. Group sharing and interaction is facilitated by regularly scheduled teleconferences. (p. 3)

DiMaria-Ghalili, et al., (2005) discussed the use of web casting technology in the graduate nursing program at West Virginia University. Web casting allows for the delivery of audio and video course content by means of the Internet. The content may be delivered synchronously and students are able to post questions that may be answered immediately by the faculty.

Skiba (2006) discussed the use of pod casting within the context of nursing education. Pod casting is "a digital recording of a radio broadcast or similar program made available on the Internet for downloading to a personal audio player." (p. 54). These devices may be used for recording and listening to lectures, listening to audio books, and other classroom related activities.

An additional method of program delivery, which is common in alternative education, is an accelerated schedule of delivery. According to Daniel (2000), "intensive or time shortened courses taught outside the traditional semester or quarter are becoming common in many colleges and universities due to the number of alternative students" (p.1).

There are many options for the delivery of alternative educational programs that are being used in nursing and other disciplines. These methods are not used exclusively in graduate programs and as such examples of undergraduate program delivery were included here. As technology continues to evolve, additional methods of alternative program delivery will likely become available.

Characteristics of Adult Learners and Related Concepts

Knowles (1996) emphasizes life experience as a key characteristic that sets the needs of adult learners apart from those of children. This experience allows the learner to be able to synthesize and attach ideas and learning concepts to issues that are pertinent their own career and life. This attachment is significant in relationship to the variety of roles that the adult learner must perform at any one given time.

Long (1990) postulated that by 1999 that the adult workers role would be "hyphenated to become the worker/learner/student role" (p. 35). This prediction did come to fruition in the context of adult students pursuing alternative graduate nursing education and advanced degrees in other fields of study.

Foundation for Adult Learning and Assumptions

Knowles, Holton, and Swanson (1998) suggest that the foundation of adult learning is based on the need of the learning to clearly understand why they need to learn information before taking on the task to do so. This is not a new concept, but is rooted in earlier work. In 1926,

Eduard C. Lindeman identified the following assumptions concerning adult learners (Lindeman, 1989):

1. Adults are motivated to learn as they experience needs and interests that learning will satisfy.
2. Adults' orientation to learning is life centered.
3. Experience is the richest source for adults' learning.
4. Adults have a deep need to be self-directing.
5. Individual differences among people increase with age.

Ostrow and DiMaria-Ghalili (2005) shared knowledge acquired about students during the process of employing distance education in a graduate nursing program:

Students are willing to learn and adapt to the various changes in distance education technology because they realize these technologies allow them the opportunity to be self directed learners. Since adults desire immediacy and application of knowledge, complete and organize information must be presented to students upfront. Detailed orientation to the technology is mandatory, so students can quickly get to the work of learning what they perceive as important in their professional goals. Discussion about the study habits needed and the differences in online courses, compared to traditional classroom instruction is essential for each class of students. (p. 9)

Prompt feedback to students is essential in distance education. Because students do not have the traditional face-to-face communication of conventional classrooms, it is vital that electronic communication be more frequent and highly responsive (p. 9).

Andragogy

The theoretical concept of andragogy (teaching of adults as opposed to children is rooted in the work of Malcolm Knowles (Knowles, et al., 1998). The andragogical learning experience

26

is learner centered and stresses personal fulfillment through a self directed learning experience. Tyler (1949) notes the following regarding the learning experience:

> The term learning experience refers to the interaction between the learning experience and the external environment to which he can react. Learning takes place through the active behavior of the student. It is what he does that he learns; not what the teacher does. (p. 63)

Paulo Freire (1993) issued a critical caution against student passivity within the context of the learning experience. "The more students work at storing the deposits entrusted in them, the less they develop the critical consciousness which would result from their intervention in the world as transformers of that world" (p. 73).

Bastable (1997) indicated that the role of the teacher in adult learning experiences is to remove obstacles that impede the process of learning or to initiate actions that enhance the process. Sinnott (1994) provided a broader description of the role by stating that:

> The classroom instructor in the andragogical model is a facilitator of learning in partnership with the learner in diagnosing the learning needs, establishing specific objectives, designing appropriate learning activities, and finally evaluating learning. (p.180)

Summary

Chapter 2 has presented a review of the literature. Historical perspectives, program delivery methods, adult learner characteristics, and the interpretive phenomenological research methodology have been explored. Chapter three will present the methodology for this study.

Chapter 3: RESEARCH METHODOLOGY

Research Design

As stated in Chapter One, the design for this study is based on similar research conducted by Mueller (2001). Mueller's research examined the phenomenon of student learning experiences in an online graduate nursing course. The participants in Mueller's study were students enrolled in an online graduate nursing course or had completed one within the prior year at a mid-western university. This study modified the examination of the phenomenon of the student learning experience by examining a sample of participants that have recently completed their graduate degree program (graduates within the last three years) and includes students from more than one university.

A qualitative interpretive phenomenological approach was utilized. Phenomenology examines the essence of a specific life experience and seeks to find the meaning of that experience (Polit, et al., 2001). The interpretive phenomenologist studies how people interpret their lives and make meaning of what they experience (Cohen, et al., 2000). The researcher actions and the ultimate goal of this methodology are appropriate to use in an attempt to answer the research questions in this study.

Restatement of the Problem

Today alternative MSN programs are accepted as the academic norm and as such are worthy of in depth examination (Ali, et al., 2004). Life circumstances, which cause students to select alternative over traditional programs and the factors they deem critical to their academic success, should be of concern to nursing programs of every variety. According to the American Association of Colleges of Nursing *White Paper* (2003), there will be more than one million vacant positions for registered nurses by 2010. Of these, 39% are positions requiring a baccalaureate or higher degree.

The issue of an aging workforce is also present in nursing academia. According to the *AACN White Paper (2003),* the national mean age of nursing faculty steadily increased over ten years (1993 to 2003) from 49.7 to 53.3 years of age for doctorally prepared and from 46 to 48.8 years of age for masters prepared faculty. The significance of these findings is directly related to the need to prepare more nursing graduates to meet the current worldwide shortage of nursing. An aging faculty workforce will result in an increase in faculty shortages due to loss of faculty members as a result of retirement. Faculty shortages serve as a stimulus for colleges and universities to consider alternative ways of educating students in order to make the most appropriate use of available resources. It is important to note that alternative educational programs will not reduce the amount of faculty workload or time commitment, but rather allow students dispersed over a larger geographic area to be taught by the same faculty, thus reducing using multiple faculty for small class groups of students.

Alternative programs for nursing education are not an isolated concept. A 2002 survey of 162 nursing programs conducted by the National League of Nursing Accrediting Commission indicated that the majority of the respondent schools were either engaged in alternative methods of instructions or had plans in to do so in the future (Ali et al., 2004).

Existing literature related to alternative MSN programs focuses on specific issues such as measurable outcomes, convenience, and accessibility. Limited attention was given to the individual student's experience or life circumstances that precipitated their choosing an alternative presentation of the curriculum Mueller (2001) stated:

> There is a growing demand for masters prepared nurses to meet the health care needs of the population. However, adult students find that multiple role responsibilities make it difficult to participate in the leisurely pace of the youth centered model of traditional higher education. (p. 1).

With this in mind, there is a need to both describe the phenomenon of the student learning experience in an alternative MSN program and understand the essence of meaning associated with this lived experience and its' impact on the student. According to Felder and Brent (2005):

> Students have different levels of motivation, different attitudes about teaching and learning, and different responses to specific classroom and instructional practices. The more thoroughly instructors understand the differences, the better chance they have of meeting the diverse needs of all their students. (p. 57)

Life experiences of student learning differ for each individual student and gaining insight into these experiences is essential in addressing the individual needs of a diverse student population.

The Purpose Statement

The purpose of the study is to explore the phenomenon of the student learning experience in an alternative Master of Science in Nursing Program in order to gain an understanding of the essence of meaning associated with this lived experience and its impact on the student. For the purpose of this study alternative refers to programs that employ methods of instruction such as online education, team learning, and/or accelerated curriculum (Kozlowski, 2002). In the same context, student learning experience refers to life circumstances that influenced the student's

30

selection of the particular alternative program and the factors that they deemed critical to academic success.

Research Questions

As stated in Chapter 1, four key research questions were used to guide this study. They were as follows:

1. What were the five primary life circumstances that influenced the decision to select an alternative MSN program over that of a traditional program?

2. What were the three major underlying themes or elements in an alternative MSN program that students deemed critical to their success?

3. What are the four primary underlying themes that facilitate a description of the overall student learning experience in an alternative MSN program?

4. What are the four primary underlying themes that facilitate a description of why the student did not select a traditional MSN program?

Sampling Procedure

The sample was purposive in nature consisting of fourteen recent graduates from three MSN programs that use alternative instructional methodology. Burns and Grove (2003) define purposive sampling as "conscious selection on the part of the researcher of certain subjects, elements, events or incidents to include in the study" (p. 255). McMillan and Schumacher (2001) refer to this technique as purposeful sampling and define it as "a strategy to choose small groups or individuals likely to be knowledgeable and informative about the phenomenon of interest; selection of cases without needing or desiring to generalize to all such cases" (p. 598).

The participants in the study had have graduated within the previous three years (2002-2005). The initial planned sample size of fifteen was an approximate number to allow researcher

31

flexibility to conduct additional interviews in order to identify additional themes to fully examine the meaning of the phenomenon or to conduct fewer depending on the outcome of initial interviews. Benner (1994) stated, "sample size is projected at the beginning of the study, but this is often adjusted depending on the quality of the text and the way that the lines of inquiry are reshaped by the participants" (p. 107).

Interview and Data Collection

Data were collected utilizing tape-recorded interviews. The interviews were transcribed verbatim. A courtroom stenographer transcribed the tapes to insure accuracy of the transcription. In addition, participants were given the opportunity to review and examine the transcript if they should request to do so.

The interview techniques utilized in this study mirrored those used by Mueller (2001). This is based on an unstructured approach. The rationale for this type of approach is to allow the participant to freely describe his/her lived experience and to allow the use of appropriate interpersonal communication techniques to bring clarification to statements made by the participant. Benner (1994) stated "because interpretive phenomenologists study every day practical knowledge and events, the communicative context is set up in naturalistic ways so that participants do not feel unduly awkward and constrained by the research interview or foreign, abstract language." (p. 108).

Before the start of the interview each participant was be informed of the purpose of the study and asked to sign the informed consent form approved by the institutional review boards of the respective interviews. Prior to the start of the interview, the participant was asked to complete a demographic data questionnaire (Appendix C). The purpose of collecting

32

demographic data is to allow the researcher to describe the sample composition and to assist in identifying any limitations brought about by the characteristics of the participants.

Interviews began with a short informal conversation in order to create a relaxed atmosphere. The participants were then asked to select a pseudonym that best suits him or her. The researcher began each interview with the following statement: "tell me a story about what the experience of learning in an alternative Master of Science in nursing was like for you." Informal open-ended questions were used during the course of the interview. The researcher sought to uncover thematic descriptions of life experiences that drew the participant to the program and specific factors that the participant deemed critical to their success. An additional example of an open-ended statement that was used is "tell me what factors you considered when deciding on an MSN program." A list of potential probative questions were developed by the researcher and used in the event of no response on the part of the participant (Appendix D). These probative questions have been designed to elicit responses in relationship to experience/behavior, opinions/values, feelings, knowledge, and the sensory experience (McMillan & Schumacher, 2001). Near the conclusion of the interview, the researcher allowed the participant the opportunity to bring clarification to specific statements made during the conversation by using open ended questions such as: Is there anything else about this experience you would like to share? Is there anything we have talked about that you would like to share further?

Content Validity of Potential Probative Questions and Demographic Questionnaire

Content validity in this study refers to demographic questionnaire and the probative questions and the extent to which they evaluate all of the major elements of the phenomenon under examination (Burns & Grove, 2003). In the context of the demographic questionnaire, this

33

refers to the ability to be able to provide a rich description of the sample composition derived from the information collected from the questionnaire. For the list of potential probative questions, this refers to the ability to obtain sufficient information and detail in order to answer the research questions posed in this study as well as uncover a core construct of meaning.

The list of probative questions and the demographic questionnaire were submitted to a panel of five doctorally prepared (PhD-2, DNSc-1, Ed.D-2) nurse educators all of whom had faculty experience in alternative nursing education as it defined in this study. Four of the five (80%) experts concurred that the demographic questionnaire would provide a rich description of the sample composition and that the list of potential probative questions would obtain sufficient information and detail in order to answer the research questions as well as identify a core construct of meaning.

Reliability

Reliability within this study refers to the degree to which the findings and conclusions derived from the study are consistent with the data collected (Merriam, 1993). Two specific strategies are employed to increase this consistency. They include triangulation by means of collection of data from three different source groups and peer examination. The purpose of peer examination is to assure that the researcher is plausibly interpreting the data and the results derived from the study are consistent with the data collected (Merriam, 1993).

Human Subjects Protection

The research proposal, informed consent and interview protocol for this study were submitted to the Pepperdine Institutional Review Board, and comparable committees from the two universities that required this. Approval was obtained and a letter of institutional permission to solicit alumni participants based upon the approval of the Pepperdine University Institutional Review Board was obtained prior to the collection of any data.

During the initial contact with the participant, the researcher confirmed that the individual met the criteria for the study explained the purpose of the study, answered any questions the participant might have, advised the participant of any risks and benefits associated with the study, and informed him or her of the option to withdraw from participation at any time. In addition, each participant was informed of the approximate time it will take for interview and data collection, methods of data analysis, and how these methods will protect confidentiality and anonymity of the participant.

All participants were asked to read and sign an informed consent form (See Appendix I). Each participant was encouraged to freely question any aspect of the research and will be provided a copy of the informed consent form. Once the individual agrees to participate in the study they were again be reminded of their option to withdraw from participation at any time.

The anonymity of participants was protected by avoiding use of names during the interview. Pseudonyms were used during the process of interview recording (Mueller, 2001). A confidential listing of code names was maintained by the researcher separate from the transcripts. The list of names and pseudonyms will be kept under lock and key. No information was included in the recorded interview or the typewritten transcript that would provide a link to the identity of the participant.

Data Analysis Procedure

Data analysis for this procedure was consistent with the interpretive phenomenological approach. Creswell (1998) described the process as follows:

The original protocols are divided into statements or horizontalization. Then the units are transformed into clusters of meanings expressed in psychological and

phenomenological concepts. Finally these transformations are tied together to make a

general description of the experience, the textural description of what was experienced,

and the structural description of how it is experienced (p.54-55).

Diekelmann, Allen, and Tanner (as cited in Polit et al., 2001) further clarified this

process by identifying seven key steps in the analysis of data within an interpretive

phenomenological study:

1. Reading all of the interviews or texts for an overall understanding.
2. Preparation of interpretive summaries of each interview.
3. Analysis of selected transcribed interviews or texts by a team of researchers.
4. Resolution of any disagreements on interpretation by going back to the text.
5. Identification of common meaning by comparing and contrasting the texts shared practices.
6. Emergence of relationships among themes.
7. Presentation of a draft of the themes, along with exemplars for the text to the team; responses and suggestions are incorporated into the final draft. (p. 393- 394)

Cohen et al. (2000) provided a practical summation of each of the steps of data analysis

within interpretive phenomenology. These steps are summarized in the following table and

served as a guide for the researcher during data analysis:

Table 1

Data Analysis Procedure

Steps in Procedure	Description
Interviews	Researcher is actively listening and thinking about the meaning of what is being said. Possible meanings for the labels may begin to be constructed.
Data Immersion	This involves reading the transcripts several times. The aim of this process is to provide an orientation to the data and an opportunity for initial interpretation that will later drive coding of the

36

	data in subsequent phases of analysis.
Data Transformation/reduction	The process is similar to editing. The researcher can reorganize the interviews placing together discussions of the same topic and eliminating digressions that are clearly off topic.
Thematic analysis	Data are examined line by line and all important phrases are labeled with tentative theme names and extract passages that have the same label that are separate from the rest of the text.
Writing and rewriting	This phase involves movement from identification and comparison of themes to a coherent picture of the whole. As the investigator gains insight and a tentative understanding of the meaning of the informant's experience, as conveyed in the exemplars and through the themes, the understandings should be summarized in written memos. These memos serve to document the hermeneutic process and drive the transformation of the field text to a coherent narrative text. (p.81-82).

Summary

This chapter describes the research design, human subjects' protection, and data analysis procedures to be used in this study. Also discussed are the sampling criteria and sampling procedures to be used. An expert panel of doctorally prepared nurse educators established content validity of both the demographic questionnaire and the potential probative questions mentioned in this chapter. Chapter four presents the analysis and key findings derived from the data.

Chapter Four: DATA ANALYSIS AND KEY FINDINGS

Introduction

Chapter three presented a description of the research methodology, human subjects'
protection, and data analysis procedure. Chapter four will present the analysis and key findings
derived from this study. The purpose of the study was to explore through formal inquiry the
phenomenon of the student learning experience in an alternative Master of Science in Nursing
Program in order to gain an understanding of the essence of meaning associated with this lived
experience and its impact on the student. Prior to presenting the analysis and key findings
derived from this study, a description of the participants will be presented.

Description of Study Participants

The purposive sample used in this study consisted of fourteen participants. Each of these
individuals was an alumnus of the three university programs included within this study. All met
the inclusion criteria of having graduated from an alternative MSN program as it defined in this
study. 13 of the participants were female and 1 was male. This was not surprising considering the
gender distribution within the realm of the nursing profession. The age of the participants ranged
between twenty-five and fifty-two with a mean age of 44.6. In terms of ethnicity, eleven of the
participants were Caucasian. The remaining three were Hispanic, Pacific Islander, and African
American.

The diversity of MSN specializations selected by the participants in this study was
somewhat narrow. Eight of the participants completed programs in nursing administration, one
completed a program with a dual specialization in administration and occupational health, three

completed generalist tracks, and two of the participants completed programs with an educator focus. None of the participants completed programs with advanced clinical practice specializations.

All of the participants were employed during the course of their alternative MSN program. The number of hours worked by each participant varied, with a mean of 34.6 hours per week. The positions held by participants were diverse and included staff positions, clinical research, and director level positions. One participant was a Certified Registered Nurse Anesthetist.

Distance of travel to class for each participant varied with a mean distance of twenty-eight miles. The frequency of required class meetings for each participant varied with a mean of 1.5. Six of the participants completed their program completely online without the necessity of traveling to campus for class meetings. The number of courses taken at one time by the participants ranged from one to four courses.

Ten of the participants were married. Eleven reported having children. One participant reported having an elderly grandfather in-law as part of her immediate family support system. For a more detailed description of the sample composition refer to Appendix J.

Overview

In order to fulfill the purpose of this study, the researcher used an interpretive phenomenological research design with non-structured interviews and a list of potential probative questions that were used in the event of no response of the part of the participants. The primary foci of this study was to gain understanding of the student learning experience within an alternative MSN program and its' impact on the student. The researcher used tape recorded interviews and verbatim transcription as an avenue to capture the participants personal

39

recollection of their lived experiences. Although some of the interview transcripts contained grammatical errors, these were not altered because doing so would change the verbatim expression and the context the comments were expressed in. Each of the transcripts was subjected to reading, rereading, and line-by-line coding. To insure plausibility of the findings a second reader was used to review the initial codes and the overall findings in order to insure consistency between the interpretation of the findings and the data that was collected. In order to triangulate the findings, participants were selected from three very different university programs. Stake (2003) described triangulation as a process of using individual perceptions of a phenomenon to clarify meaning and different ways in which the phenomenon is being seen.

Analysis and Key Findings Derived from the Study

Four research questions served as the guide for the inquiry. This section will present the key themes emerging from the participant interviews in relationship to each of the four research questions as well as pointed exemplars from the interview transcripts that substantiate the existence of these themes. The truths revealed by each of the participants have been considered equally in this process without regard to the particular MSN program that they graduated from.

Identification of key themes and pointed exemplars from the participant interviews was less than an easy process. The fourteen participant interviews yielded in excess of 250 pages of verbatim transcript, all of which was subjected to in depth examination. This examination brought for the themes and exemplars in response to the four research questions in this study.

Research Question #1

Research Question #1 asks: *What are the five primary life circumstances that influenced the decision to select an alternative MSN program over that of a traditional program?* Although this question seeks to uncover five themes, only three emerged from the participant interviews.

40

The following themes emerged from the participant interviews in relationship this question: *Moving on, competing family responsibilities, and long commute.* The following paragraphs will include supporting exemplars in relationship to each of three themes identified.

During the course of graduate study, life circumstances continue to evolve and may include *moving on* either to a new place of employment or to a new geographic area. The following key exemplars share the story of participants who relocated during the course of graduate study:

> Elizabeth Stated: I wouldn't be able to move. What I was able to do was move out to a different state in order to complete the last quarter of my program, the residency. And because of the online course, I was able to do that residency out of state. There was one course that I had to complete at the same time of doing this project, or projects. There was no way I could have completed that course in a classroom setting and then also, at the same time, 3,000 miles away, completed a residency.

Gloria shared a similar experience in that her alternative MSN program allowed her to have exposure to a variety of states by means of doing her program practicum work with a nationwide consulting firm. This multi-state exposure led to her permanent relocation to the east coast upon graduation. Gloria said:

> The last quarter, the last two quarters -- actually, the last semester -- was when we did our program and we were able to select an area that we chose. So I chose consulting. So -- and I was able to travel and do my online classroom time from wherever. I traveled to Montana; I traveled to Portland Oregon -- time then. It was changed where you only had to go to class -- was in town, I would go to classroom.

41

So what I did while I was in school was the case management redesign, which was the last semester, and then they also let me go with the different consultants on the different projects they were out. So they would go -- we went to Illinois --and I can't remember the city right now. But we went to Illinois and they were looking at going in there and doing an assessment of what it was that that particular hospital wanted.

The majority of participants discussed the challenges of balancing work and family commitments. *Competing family responsibilities* were seen as significant within the process of selecting an alternative MSN program. Many times these responsibilities extend far beyond what one would normally perceive. Ray stated:

> I have two daughters that have severe bipolar disorder. And I was carrying a full load, I like 16 credit hours, and working full-time and my daughters were in and out of the hospital, and I couldn't do it. It was too intense for me. So I -- I kept looking for something else and I checked out the university and I was intrigued by it.
>
> My husband, he tried to sidetrack the kids as much as possible. But I -- he felt   very isolated because I would be penned up in my den from like 4:00 o'clock in the afternoon till way past 12 midnight many, many nights. And so we didn't mostly have a whole -- we didn't have a real enriching lifestyle during that time because I was pretty dedicated to school.

Ray was most certainly not alone in her struggle to balance family responsibilities. Gina shared the experience of having a child during her graduate program and anticipating doing so when she started the program. Gina said:

> There was a portion of the – at the beginning of the master's program, I did; I was pretty much with the same students. But I was – you know, ended up deciding to have

a child right in the middle of it. So when I had my son, I skipped one course and took I guess it was six weeks off and that put me into a class with new students.

Brittany also iterated the challenges of balancing home life, school and work responsibilities. Brittany stated:

A very tight schedule, extremely tight schedule: From work to home, study, having to negotiate at work a lot to get time off, try to go -- drive to the university and then I had to drive back to work again. So that was a little bit stressful.

The issue of *long commute* times in relationship to program selection was no surprise considering that the mean distance of travel for each of the participants in this study was 27.8 miles. Puffs noted:

Um, I had a long commute and because of the long commute, I was very glad to have the online course -- courses available to me because it really cut down the hours I had to spend -- wasted hours in that sense.

It's really funny when I first started there, my first quarter I had many, many classes. And initially I tried driving back and forth every day, but I brought this old clunker of an RV and actually stayed overnight in the parking lot 'cause I had classes all day Monday and Monday night and the early morning Tuesday. So I'd drive up Sunday night, after I'd finish working, and I might leave home here sometime between 10:00 and midnight and arrive on campus in the parking lot sometime between midnight and 3:00 a.m. and sleep for a little bit and then get up and go into class and then have a few classes and then come back and eat my supper, and then I had a class that evening sometimes and then same thing again the next day. So that – that was interesting. So that was like Monday and Tuesday. So I'd leave Sunday night, Monday and Tuesday. And then on

Thursday and Friday, I would have classes as well. But they were always on ground

because some of them were at site visits, so it might be anywhere in Southern California.

And that was tough, too, because I'd have to get up -- well, a lot of times if I had to go to

campus I'd leave at 3:00 in the morning. So it was a real relief for me to be online when I

didn't have to do that as constantly. It was really tough. I was exhausted.

Mark concurred that distance was an issue that became integral to attempt the alternative
portion of his MSN program. Mark said:

For me it was distance. I was probably the one of two people who was not -- or one of

three people who was not at the current, you know, the university region, the--county

region. So, you know, going to school, driving 60 miles one way back and forth for two

to three times a week was a selling point. And, you know, them saying it's flexible. I've

tried other online programs before. So sure, it was a no-brainer at that point.

A long commute is not an isolated concept to those who talk about it. It is

important to note that 6 of the participants completed their program in a virtual format

and although a long commute was not specifically mentioned by them as an issue in

regard to program selection it is certainly worthy of consideration.

Research Question # 2

Research Question #2 asks: *What were the three underlying themes or elements in*

alternative MSN program that students deem critical to their success? The following themes

emerged from the participant interviews in relationship to this research question: *Professional*

Connections, open channels of communication, and intrinsic desire and motivation. The

following paragraphs will include supporting exemplars in relationship to each of the three

themes.

The importance of *professional connections* in relationship to academic success was expressed by the majority of the participants. These professional connections varied in type and were inclusive of fellow students, faculty, and outside mentors and experts.

Victoria pointed out that professional connections facilitate the process of students learning from one another:

> Well, I think one of the things that actually became one of the best things about it was the opportunity to interact with nurses all over the country and see both the differences and the similarities in our working experiences, um, and to also have instructors that were from all over the country. And, you know, some people lived in large cities, some people were very rural, and we came from all different clinical experiences. So it just led to just such wonderful discussions about whatever the topic of the week was.

Gloria described her experience of withdrawal and reentry to her graduate program and how her professional connection with a particular faculty provided support for her and encouraged her to return:

> Um, actually, I had started the program a year prior to my actually going in. What had happened was I had been accepted into the program, went into the program, and my husband was laid off from his job two weeks into the program. So I had to quit. And of course, we were really upset. He had been with this company for 20 years and was laid off. So (name deleted) from the university called me at home and talked to me for a long time, and then I think she called one other time six months later just to check on me. That was actually what led me to know that that was absolutely the program that I wanted to go back into.

Molly shared the tremendous reward that she obtained from professional connections during her graduate program and the learning and sharing opportunities it provided her:

I had the interaction with other nurses and then we -- we, throughout the program, had online assignments and we had a chat group, you know, where we'd do projects together. And we would work online and then we would get together in the classroom setting once or twice a week and I loved the combination. I loved having the relationships and meeting people and building relationships and friendships and mentoring, because being the older nurse in the class and just having, you know, 29 years of nursing experience. We had a wide range of people who were in the program, but it was really very rewarding to be with nurses that really looked up to myself.

Molly shared information about the diversity and professional connections within her class and how these contributed to her learning experience and success as a result of the support it provided:

Um, all different nationalities -- you know, Vietnamese and Hispanic and Caucasian -- and all different career paths. Lots of different experiences: People who worked for the Public Health Department, people who worked in home health, people who worked in the hospital. So every kind of background and experiences, male and female. A pretty small, intimate group. You know, we weren't a large group of nurses, maybe 20 or 25 of us; the instructors were friendly and welcoming and tried to help us be at ease; a sense of excitement and a sense of, oh, my gosh so -- and it was really great having like a best friend to go through the experience together for support.

Professional connections are integral to the second theme identified as critical to the

success of the participants. *Open channels of communication* were identified as an essential

factor to a large portion of the participants in this study. Marci Duffy shared how open channels

of communication with her faculty led to her being able to successfully complete the required

practicum course that was a part of her MSN program:

> It was great. We actually had telephone conversation even after the program because we
>
> did practicum one and practicum two. So after the class completed, we still have to keep
>
> in touch with the faculty in order to transition into practicum two. So we did a lot of
>
> phone conversation, e-mailing and not just posting. But she was very, very supportive
>
> and that helped. very helpful because we have like, you know, four columns. So we did
>
> column one, we send it in. We got feedback from that in column two. Then, you know,
>
> feedback from that in column three and then the final one for column four. So, you
>
> know, for the final project, you know, it's practically perfect because you already get all
>
> the feedback, you know, throughout the course.

Sally described how open channels of communication between she and her

classmates contributed to the learning of the group:

> It was really, really an important part of -- of my learning, because you have people from
>
> all parts of the United States in all fields of nursing and we would feed off of each other,
>
> you learn so much from each other. You quickly learn that your viewpoint depends on
>
> which area of nursing you're working in at the time.

Mark provided a very different description of his experience that illustrates the

consequences when *open channels of communication* are not present or become

dysfunctional:

47

They gave an assignment, maybe three or four questions. You had to assign those -- you

had to answer those questions and then respond to a couple of members of your group to

consider an assignment for that week to complete. Well, that's where the flexibility issue

comes in, because it actually isn't flexible because my schedule may not necessarily be

my colleague's schedule. So if they decide to finish their part of their assignments on the

sixth day, which I may not have time to do, I can't necessarily get my piece in place to

complete my assignment.

Puffs shared how *open channels of communication* can become compromised

when what is written in an online discussion is not interpreted the same way it was

intended:

Well, sometimes, you know, we'd have a discussion, a threaded discussion, and

sometimes I'd respond back and acknowledge what was said and then sort of give a "yes,

but" portion of it and "what do you think of" to try to get my question, what I was really

seeking, out there. And it turned reverse as well, because when I would be posting

something as part of the discussion, people would not always understand the

communication that I was sending out. So it was interesting to learn how people

responded to what you wrote as opposed to what you meant.

In addition to *professional connections and open channels of*

communication, intrinsic motivation was also described by many of the participants as critical to

their success during the process of graduate study. Brittany shared her perceptions regarding the

need intrinsic motivation and self- discipline in order to be successful in graduate study:

You have to be very rigid with time management. You have to set schedules. Nobody is

watching over your back. You have to learn on your own. You don't have somebody, a professor there. And you're not in a class to be asking so many questions or things like that. But the most important thing is independent study. And you have to be able to because of the response I get from a lot of people, "Well, I've been out of school for so many years" -- five, six, ten, 15 years -- "I don't see myself studying without an instructor or in the class." That's the response I get from everyone: I do not see myself doing that; it's impossible.

Molly agreed and she shared how intrinsic motivation fed her drive for exemplary academic achievement. Molly said:

I think a lot of internal motivation and, like I said, I really put 150 percent into it where my friend, she had a much more relaxed attitude about it and I had like this total high achiever attitude and wanting to just, you know, do everything like A, you know. And I accomplished that, you know. I just – I put a lot of extra pressure on myself because I wanted to just really achieve. I had an internal thing, so --.

Sally shared how her intrinsic motivation drove her to exceed course requirements by taking on a "have to" attitude to engage in daily course participation:

You have -- you have to just say, I'm going to be in that classroom every day. The only day I might have skipped would be Thursday, when the new week started. But other than that, I went there every day.

Sparky described how intrinsic motivation kept her engaged and maintained her Momentum to keep her in graduate school:

Sheer perseverance, that's all. I was thinking about that the other night when I was talking to my friend and she kept saying, "I'm amazed that you could do as much as you did." And you just -- you do it. You just do it. You have to have the goal in mind. The

49

first half of any program, I don't care what you're doing, the first half you could quit. You know, it's easy to quit. But once you crossed the point of no return, which is you started the second half, if you quit now, you've lost. Whereas if you keep trudging through, you have everything to gain and nothing to lose.

Research Question # 3

Research Question #3 asks: *Which four underlying themes facilitate a description of the overall learning experience in an alternative MSN program?* The following key themes in relationship to this research question: New and alternative opportunities for learning, formalized and focused discussion, frustration, and not for everyone.

New and alternative opportunities for learning emerged as a key theme in relationship to the learning experience for many of the participants. Gina shared her perceptions regarding new and alternative learning opportunities in the online environment:

I could go sit in a classroom and it could go in one ear and out the other, but because I'm present in a classroom that means I'm learning? I don't know. I don't really buy into that. I think people learn different ways and it's just different perception. It's nontraditional, you know, and it's getting more and more and people are, I think, using it more. But I don't think you have to be present in a room with a teacher to learn.

Brittany identified how the online learning environment created an expanded opportunity outside of the traditional classroom to enhance her writing skills. She said:

Well, I'm going to be very honest. Something that was of a great, great significance to me with my experience online was the fact that my writing skills increased drastically because with online, I had to write a lot more than just writing one or two papers and turning them for the entire semester or writing one semester one paper for the whole semester and having maybe one multiple choice question. It was not like that. Now I was writing and writing every two days, every three days and answering.

Sherry talked about the broad learning opportunities available within her alternative MSN program and how she narrowed her focus. She said:

You know, I learned about the financials of my hospital, the whole PI program, the research aspects, just so much. I learned how to create a business plan. So there's just so many options that would be out there for me, and I focused more on the research aspect 'cause that's where my focus is.

Ray how her program afforded her the learning opportunity to look beyond her role as a busy CRNA and see a broader picture of the nursing profession:

I have to tell you that being a nurse anesthetist, I'm speaking -- I'm generalizing here – I think that we get so narrow-minded in that way. We have tunnel vision and we think that we're the best, you know. And we're in the operating room and we're behind the drapes, and we think that the patient -- we're the

only important person taking care of that patient, that anesthesia is the most important role. And it's not that operating room nurse has got so much that they give that they bring to the team, and I think a log of us, we forget that we're part of the team.

I didn't appreciate, um, what risk management does. You know, I didn't really have a good handle on what quality assurance was. That program with the university, I -- I got so many -- it's like looking at a 12-lead EKG.

Formalized and focused discussion was a very clear theme across the participant interviews in terms of describing the learning experience in relationship to classroom interaction. Gloria talked about the need to be prepared for these discussions:

> What I found was it really made you do your homework. You couldn't just fake it. Like, if you would go to class, even if you were tired, you can sit there and not necessarily interact with people.

Elizabeth agreed regarding the focus on classroom content in the discussion and little room to discuss anything else. She said:

> I recall all the threaded discussion being required. I don't recall us actually needing to discuss anything outside of, like, an assignment. I believe we had threaded discussion assignments where we had to, um, discuss something or accomplish something through that threaded discussion forum.

Brittany shared a very similar response and emphasized the importance of incorporating appropriate conceptual support while engaging in the classroom discussion. This did not occur initially She stated:

> It was -- for the questions you had to --at the very beginning, like I said, everybody was just answering like, "Oh, I feel" -- the questions were not backed up by -- by our resources which was our theory, our content that we were learning. People were just answering as they went along based on experience. So we were told that that wasn't the purpose of the discussion. When we discuss something, we have to have backup for it which, once again, our textbooks, our content, our theory. That's the way we need to respond.

Victoria shared how her program focused the student on course at a time, concentrating on one particular area of content. She stated:

> But thinking about taking, you know, four or, you know, four classes each semester
> and trying to do an entire program in the time I did it, traditional versus online, being
> able to take it one class at a time, focus on that even though it was six weeks, to me
> was just -- it was so much easier. I was able to just focus my attention onto that class,
> understand it, learn from it or, you know, just get myself through it, depending on what
> class it was, like health care finance.

In spite of new and alternative learning opportunities, formalized and focused discussion, *frustration* did surface for a good number of the participants. Sherry shared how group work and the dishonest act of a classmate led to her frustration:

> The group work was my major frustration. I liked the idea of evaluating your teammates
> because I really don't think it's fair if someone does, you know, really inferior work – you
> know, I had one girl on my team with a group paper, we each had to write a segment of
> it, and her whole paper was plagiarized, word for word. Yeah. So, you know, we couldn't
> use that. And this paper was due and she turned it in at the last minute, you know, like a
> few hours before it's done. Well, you know, we had to scramble and we missed the
> deadline, and then she ended up with the same grade as we did. So that was very
> frustrating.

Marci Duffy also identified group work to be a source of frustration. She said:

> I'm going to give you an experience here. We did a research paper. And it was supposed
> to be a quantitative research, but -- we thought it was a quantitative research, but it
> wasn't. It was a qualitative research. So we did it, you know. I mean, we did it and we

sent it in like two hours before deadline. Lo and behold, the instructor sent back to say we did not do a quantitative research, we did a qualitative research. My team members were all happy and gone. But I'm a late person, so I was on the computer. And she gave us a chance to redeem ourselves or else we were going to get a zero on the paper. And I had to do that paper all by myself, because they were all gone, everybody was just happy. But I'm a person I like to log on, you know, late at night, 3:00 o'clock in the morning. So I'd log on. And the next day I called them and we talk and, you know, it was like, okay, everyone was happy, but I had to do that all by myself. And that was the worst time in my life in that program.

Mark identified his source of frustration within the learning experience to be communication. Mark stated:

The frustrating part, where I was frustrated at, was having to wait for a response from my colleagues. And, you know, the selling point of the online program, seeing it was a, you know, online it was supposed to be a flexible program, which I believed it wasn't because of the way they had that formatting.

Sparky identified initial frustration of being in the online learning environment that was very temporary in nature for a negative source of frustration into a positive experience. She said:

Well, part of my classes were online. And the experience initially was a negative one; I didn't like the idea of not being in the classroom. But I found that being online and being able to do classes online and course work online was actually very freeing because you don't have to face other people, you simply have to interact with them in a different media.

The participants in the study repeatedly stated that an alternative MSN program is *not for everyone.* Elizabeth shared her thoughts regarding this:

> So I think for that reason with online learning you really have to be self-disciplined and
> know how to break down things to bite-sized sizes so you can get
> -- you know, accomplish things. You can't wait till the last minute. And I think some
> people just aren't cut out for that.

Victoria had very similar comments to Elizabeth. She compared the learning process to a road map. She said:

> No, it's not for everyone. You know, you have to be really self directed. You have to be
> very disciplined. It's really easy to fall off the map on it, you know. But I'm going, they
> were really great classes and, yeah, you make it what you want to be.

Sally further reinforced that an alternative MSN program may not be the best option for many students due to time requirements and the necessary of personal commitment. She stated:

> Yeah, I would caution students definitely caution students
> about the fact that online education takes an immense amount of time. It takes much,
> much dedication. I think online education is harder, it's more challenging, it takes a lot of
> you as a person to be able to do it. And if you don't feel that you can spend six hours, you
> know, a day or four hours a day doing it, then don't start because you don't have that
> luxury. You can't just skip class.

Ray commented about the need for adaptation to the online environment. She said "it's a different type of learning and it's something that I adapted to." Adaptation does not occur for every student and as such this type of learning environment is *not for everyone.*

Research Question #4

Research Question #4 asks: *What are the four primary underlying themes that facilitate a description why the students did not select a traditional MSN program?* The following themes emerged from the participant interviews in relationship to this research question: Flexibility and choice, extreme distance, reviewability, and focused delivery.

Flexibility and choice emerged in all of the participant interviews Each of the participants described this concept in a slightly different way. Puffs talked about the advantage of being able to choose the time and place for learning to occur. She said:

Flexibility is wonderful because you can do it in your pajamas at midnight or whatever time works in your life. So the flexibility is really nice and it's very comfortable surroundings when you're in your own home. It's not like you're sitting in the chair in school and that may or may not be the most comfortable part.

Elizabeth agreed. She said "I have a computer and I have the internet access. So I was able to complete the course during a time that was convenient for me."

Marci Duffy talked about how *flexibility and choice* permitted her to complete her education while continuing to work full time. She said:

The convenience; that's, you know, time I can work and go to school full-time and -- really the convenience and also the experience with working with -- going to school with adults. And the learning experience was great.

Molly talked about the applicability of her course content directly to her work and the flexibility of choosing her own learning environment. Molly stated:

So make maybe it was leadership in theory, but you could apply it in any way you chose. So that was really, really exciting about the program. Because everything I learned I could apply at work. And so much of the learning that I was doing I was applying right here on the job and I implemented programs and I did so much real-life implementation of things through my studies.

Flexibility doe not always rest in staying in an alternative MSN program. Mark had very different comments concerning flexibility and choice in that flexibility for him meant the option to return to the traditional classroom environment. He said:

Um, like I said, I was only probably there for, you know, a few assignments from what I recall. And, you know, I -- from my, you know, from my demographics and, you know, the needs I need to put into my family, you know, I can either -- it just wasn't worth it to have to manipulate your time in a seven-day period. Why do that when I can just go to class one day a week, two days a week, X amount and I could plan a little better for those days and be done with versus a variable seven days, give or take, each week? I don't know.

The issue of distance to attend emerged in the first research question, but it also surfaced in terms of the reason why the participant chose not to attend a traditional MSN program. *Extreme distance* was one factors considered by many of the participants. Victoria said "I was traveling like an hour and a half a couple of times a week just to go to school. Gloria stated "I drove ninety miles one way to school." Puff had similar comments she said: "

Um, I had a long commute and because of the long commute, I was very glad to have the

online course -- courses available to me because it really cut down the hours I had to

spend -- wasted hours in that sense.

Reviewability surfaced as a descriptor in many of the participant interviews as why

a traditional MSN program was not selected. In the context of this discussion, *reviewability*

refers to the option to return to classroom content and discussions to review them at a later date

or time. Puffs shared how reviewability in the online environment was advantageous to her. She

said:

I really valued the online part because it's there, it's permanent, you can access it again;

whereas when you're in a classroom, you have your notes to go to or any readings that

were given, but you don't have any of the discussion available to you easily. And that

was a true advantage.

Marci Duffy shared similar comments about being able to review the content at a later

date. She said:

I could go back days after, months after and look back through all the postings, read

everything that's there, print it out if you want and, you know, get more information from

that. And the classroom, when it's done, it's done.

In addition to *reviewability, focused delivery* was also an important factor to many of

the participants. Ray said: "I liked the fact that you only take one class at a time. It was very

intense, but it was one class at a time." Victoria stated:

But thinking about taking, you know, four or, you know, four classes each semester and

trying to do an entire program in the time I did it, traditional versus online, being able to take it one class at a time, focus on that even though it was six weeks, to me was just --it was so much easier.

Sherry had very similar comments concerning focused delivery in her graduate program. She said:

> You can focus on one class at a time. You can really focus your energy on learning that, you know, learning all the concepts of that, all the papers you're writing, all the research you're doing, questions that you're answering, it's all on one subject.

Seeking a Core Construct of Meaning

The act of obtaining answers the four research questions above would be limiting from an interpretive phenomenological perspective without uncovering a core construct of meaning regarding the lived experience of the participants. The core construct of meaning threaded in each of the participant interviews is *uplifting*. This lived experience has been uplifting to the participants in terms of new professional opportunities, increased self confidence, and a new direction in life. The following exemplars illustrate how this experience has been *uplifting* to the participants in this study.

> Puffs: It's been life changing, totally life changing. I still pinch myself. I can't believe this has happened to me. I'm having a really hard time not going back for my Ph.D.

> Elizabeth: It's meant being able to get an advanced degree, and I wouldn't certainly be in the position I am now being able to have a -- at my current role I have a global scope. I wouldn't be in the position to be qualified for that role if it wasn't for my advanced degree.

Brittany: It has a lot of meaning to me. It has a tremendous meaning to me because going through graduate school, I'm the first one and the only one in my family who's ever been to college. So that alone -- I don't know if it's a challenge or not, but it was different. I'm the only one that has a college degree.

Victoria: It gave me the tools and worked on my strengths and allowed me to develop my weaknesses into strengths so that I could do that effectively. And I felt like I just kept building on that and then, you know, I moved into my postgraduate degree to get my clinical nurse specialist, and education is still a big part of that.

Gloria: It would have -- well, the whole administrative world was new to me. I had always been a staff nurse, never even gone into the management. I had been charge nurse, but not anything higher than that level. And it's just – the university, you know, really helped me be prepared more than I even imagined, because now I feel really comfortable just walking into the CEO's

office, CFO's office, whatever. I think it just really helped my comfort level knowing what to expect.

Sparky: Um, I guess if I was going to say anything about the entire experience, it would be it was a life-changing experience and not just to get the letters behind my name.

MOLLY: Um, it's been very valuable to me. Like I

said in the beginning, it really -- seeking new knowledge I think really expands your horizons. It just kind of opens up the world much broader. So learning does, I think it opens our perspective and our and our understanding of the world. I felt very successful in my graduate study so I think it helped to develop a greater sense of confidence and a sense of accomplishment, esteem to having gone through this level.

Sally: Professionally, it has taken me to a level of nursing I never thought I would see. And my greatest pleasure now is I work in the school district. And where I work, nurses were somewhere down on the food chain with -- janitors were more important. The nurses -- to them, to this school district, nurses were a necessary evil. They got no respect, nobody wanted to deal with them. And in the last year I have been able to raise the profession of nursing in this school district to a level that they are held in high regard with great respect. And that is what this profession to me is all about. To be able to see these school nurses rise up like that has been awesome. And personally, I'm a completely different person than the person that started grad school. Much more confident, excited, excited about learning, excited about using my knowledge. And not just -- not limited to nursing, but to anything in my life. You know, you walk six feet taller.

Lolita: Well, means to me I had a bit of kind of sort of is that I'm a good example to my children. I have four daughters, and one has – two have finished college, one is in college, one is starting college. So I'm trying to be a good example to my own children and letting them know, number one, that education is important. Number two, that you can achieve whatever you want to if you just set your mind to it. That it's never too late to go back to school no matter how old you are. You can always do it. It's not, you know, that intimidating. Go for it.

Summary

Chapter four has presented a description of the study participants, research questions, themes and exemplars in response to each research question, and a core construct of meaning the participants' lived experience in an alternative MSN program. Chapter Five will include implications and directions for further research.

CHAPTER 5: IMPLICATIONS AND DIRECTIONS FOR FURTHER RESEARCH

Implications

Alternative graduate nursing education continues to proliferate and new methods of program delivery are being developed at a pace exceeding that of research. The positive impact of these types of programs on the lives of students is supported by the core construct of meaning (uplifting) revealed in this study. Reality is non-static and individualistic in nature and as such so is the meaning of the lived experience of graduate study for each student (Streubert-Speziale & Carpenter, 2007). Further formal inquiry in regards the student's lived experience of learning is needed in order to understand that experience in the context of current technology.

This research provides important information regarding the study participants' lived experience of student learning, the factors that they deem critical to critical to their success, and essential information related to rationale as to why the students' chose traditional versus alternative graduate nursing education. It is important to remember that these lived experiences are subjective in nature are reflective of the participant's personal recollection of that experience.

Potential implications stemming from this research include providing guidance to reduce learner frustrations in alternative instructional programs, as well as best practices identification of specific best practices that student's deem critical to their academic success. These are worthy of consideration, but should also be scrutinized prior to application in other educational settings.

Recommendations for Further Research

This study by no means explores the lived experience of alumni from every type of every type of masters' graduate nursing program that uses alternative instructional methodology as defined in this study. It is essential that additional research be conducted in regards to this experience in advanced clinical practice programs that incorporate this type of instruction.

Masters degree programs in nursing are not the only type of graduate nursing program that currently incorporates alternative instructional methodology. Doctoral programs in nursing are also following suit and as such the lived experience in an alternative doctoral program in nursing is an important target area for future research efforts.

In addition to the exploration of lived experience, it is worthy to consider the use of quantitative research methodology in order to examine the proliferation and student enrollment in these types of graduate nursing programs. A coherent picture of volume and magnitude is essential to provide background and significance data for future research efforts.

Summary

The alternative graduate nursing arena will continue to grow and as such research must continue in order to maintain a current and comprehensive understanding of that lived experience. This study explored the lived experience of fourteen participants who completed their education during a specified time period. Reality is not static nor can the efforts be to maintain a current and comprehensive understanding of students' educational experiences. This study is merely the beginning of a lifetime research agenda attempting to maintain a current understanding of the "lived experience of student learning."

REFERENCES

Ali, N.S., Hodson-Carlton, K., & Ryan, M. (2004). Student perceptions of online learning: Implications for teaching. *Nurse Educator, 29*(3), 111-115.

American Association of Colleges of Nursing (2003). *White Paper: Faculty shortages in Baccalaureate and graduate nursing programs: Scope of the problem and strategies for expanding the supply.* Retrieved June 14th, 2004 from http://www.acn.nhe.edu/Publications/White Papers/Faculty Shortages.htm

Appleton, J.V. & King, L. (1997). Constructivism: A naturalistic inquiry. *Advances in Nursing Science, 20*(2), 13-22.

Bastable, S.B. (1997). *Nurse as educator: Principles of teaching and learning.* Subury, MA: Jones and Bartlett Publishers.

Bates, A.W. & Poole, G. (2003). *Effective teaching with technology in higher education: Foundations for Success* (1st ed.). San Francisco, CA: John Wiley & Sons.

Benner, P. (1994). The tradition and skill of interpretive phenomenology in studying health, illness and caring practices. In P. Benner (Ed.). *Interpretive phenomenology: Embodiment, caring, and ethics in health and illness (p. 108).* Thousand Oaks, CA: Sage.

Bogie, B. & Gilbert, C. (2005). Elluminate delivers real-time interaction to Australia's Deakin University; Live eLearning environment will also provide support for off-campus Students, cross-campus meetings, and professional development for teachers and staff. *Business Wire.* July 19, 2005, p. 1.

Brogdon, L.M., & Couros, A. (2002). Contemplating the virtual campus: Pedagogical and administrative considerations. *Delta Kappa Gamma Bulletin, 68*(3), 22-30.

Brownson, K. & Harriman, R.L. (2000). Distance education in the twenty-first century. *Hospital*
    Material Management Quarterly, 22(2), 64-69.

Burns, N. & Grove, S.K. (1997). *The practice of nursing research: Conduct, critique, and*
    *utilization (*3rd ed.). Philadelphia: W.B. Saunders.

Burns, N. & Grove, S.K. (2003). *Understanding nursing research* (3rd ed.). Philadelphia: W.B.
    Saunders.

Carter, L. (2003). Distance wise reflection for Ontario Nursing. *The Canadian Nurse, 99*(10), 1-
    7.

Cohen, M.Z., Kahn, D.L., & Steeves, R.H. (2000). *Hermeneutic phenomenological research: A*
    practical guide for nurse researchers. Thousand Oaks, CA: Sage.

Costello, B. Lenholt, R. & Stryker, J. (2004). Using Blackboard in library instruction.
    Addressing the learning styles of Generation X and Y. *Journal of Academic*
    Librarianship, 30(6). 452-460.

Creswell, J.W. (1998). *Qualitative inquiry and research design: Choosing among the five*
    traditions. Thousand Oaks, CA: Sage.

Daniel, E.L. (2000). A review of time-shortened courses across disciplines. *College Student*
    Journal, 34(2), 298-308.

Denzin. N.K. & Lincoln, L.S. (1994). *Handbook of qualitative research.* Thousand Oaks, CA:
    Sage.

DiMaria-Ghalili, R.A., Ostrow, L., & Rodney, K. (2005). Webcasting: A new instructional
    technology in graduate nursing education. *Journal of Nursing Education, 44*(1). 11-17.

Felder, R.M. & Brent, R. (2005). Understanding student differences. *Journal of Engineering*
    Education, 94(1). 57-72.

Fraenkel, J.R. & Wallen, N.E. (2001). *Educational research: A guide to the process.* Mahwah,
   NJ: Lawrence Earlbaum Associates.

Freire, P. (1993). *Pedagogy of the Oppressed.* New York: Continuum International Publishing
   Inc.

George, L. (2002). E-Communities in Distance Learning. *Library Mosaics,* 14-16.

Giorgi, A. (1985). *Phenomenology and psychological research.* Pittsburgh, PA: Duquesne
   University Press.

Heidegger, M. (1962). *Being and time.* San Francisco, CA: Harper Collins Publishers.

Higher Education Reports (2002). *Quality in distance learning.* Retrieved March 20th, 2004
   from http://80 vnweb.hwwilsonweb.com.lib.pepperdine.edu/hwww/resulty/results
   _single.jhtml?nn

Hogan, P. (n.d.) *Hermeneutics and educational experience.* Retrieved January 23rd , 2005 from
   http://www.vusst.hr/Encyclopaedia/her.htm

Hoy, D. (1985). This critical circle: Literature, history, and philosophical hermeneutics. In K.
   Mueller-Vollmer (Ed), *The hermeneutics reader.*

Jeffries, P. (2005). Technology trends in nursing education: Next Steps. *Journal of Nursing
   Education, 44*(1), 3-4.

Johnson, S. & Romanello, M.L. (2005). Generational Diversity: teaching and learning
   approaches. *Nurse educator, 30*(5), 212-216.

Kay, A. (1995). *The virtual campus: Technology and reform in higher education.* Washington,
   DC: Educom.

Knowles, M.S., Holton, E.F., & Swenson, R.A. (1998) *The adult learner* (5th ed.). Houston, TX:
   Gulf Publishing Company.

Knowles, M. (1996). Adult learning. In R.L. Craig (Ed), *The ASTD training and development handbook* (pp. 253-293). New York, NY: McGraw Hill.

Kozlowski, D. 2002). Returning to school: An alternative to traditional education. *Orthopaedic Nursing, 21*(4), 47.

Levin, S.R., Levin, J.A., Buell, J.G., & Waddoups, G.L., (2002). Curriculum, technology, and education reform (CTER) online. Evaluation of an online master of education program. *Tech trends, 46*(3), 1-11.

Lindeman, E.C. (1989). *The meaning of adult education.* New York: Harvest House Printing.

Long, H.B. (1990). Understanding adult learners. In M.W. Gailbrath (Ed), *Adult learning methods.* Malabar, FL: Krieger Publishing Company.

Lopez, K.A. & Willis, D.G. (2004). Descriptive versus interpretive phenomenology: Their contributions to nursing knowledge. *Qualitative Health Research, 14* (5). 726-765.

Lorenzo, G. (2003). Hybrid structure offers flexibility to working students. *Distance Education Report, 7*(3), 5.

McMillan, J.M. & Schumacher, S. (2001). *Research in education* (5th ed.). New York: Addison Wesley Longman, Inc.

Merriam, S.B. (1993). *What can you tell from an N of 1?* Issues of validity and reliability in qualitative research. Retrieved June 27, 2005 from http://www.coe.uga.edu/quig/merriam93.html

Merriam, S.B. & Caffarella, R.S. (1999). *Learning in adulthood* (2nd ed.). San Francisco: Jossey-Bass.

Mueller, C.L., (2001). Masters in nursing student's experiences as a member of a virtual classroom on the internet. *Book Abstracts International., 62*(08) p. 3557 (ISBN No. 0-493-36038-7).

Ostrow, L. & DiMaria-Ghallili, (2005). Distance education. one state school's experience. *Journal of Nursing Education, 44*(1), 5-9.

Polit, D.F., Beck, C.T., & Hungler, B.P., (2001). *Essentials of nursing research: Methods, appraisal, and utilization* (5th ed.). Philadelphia: Lippincott.

Sinnott, J.D., (1994). *Interdisciplinary handbook of adult and lifespan learning.* Westport, CN: Greenwood Press.

Skiba, D., (2006). Emerging technologies center: The 2005 Word of the year: Podcast. *Nursing Education Perspectives, 27*(1), 54-55.

Solomon, J.L., (1987). *From Hegel to existentialism.* New York: Oxford University Press.

Stake, R., (2003). Case Studies. In N.K. Denzin & Y.S. Lincoln (Eds). *Strategies of qualitative inquiry* (pp. 134-164). Thousand Oaks, CA: Sage Publications.

Streubert-Speziale, H.J. & Rinaldi-Carpenter, D., (2007). *Qualitative research in nursing: Expanding the humanistic imperative.* Philadelphia: Lippincott, Williams & Wilkins.

Sykes, S.A. (2003). U. live video school teaches PhD in nursing nationwide. *Salt Lake Tribune.* July 15, 2003, p. 2-3.

Tisdell, E., (1999). Adult education philosophy informs practice. *Adult learning, 11*, 6.

Tyler, R.W. (1949). *Basic principles of curriculum and instruction.* Chicago, IL: University of Chicago Press.

Van Manen, M. (1990). *Researching lived experiences: Human sciences for action sensitive pedagogy.* Albany, NY: State University of New York Press.

Wagschal, K. (1997). I became clueless teaching the Gen Xers: Redefining the profiles of the adult learner. *Adult Learning. 8*, 21-25.

Wambach, K., Boyle, D. Hagemaster, J., Teel, C., Langner, B., Fazzone, P. et al. (1999). Beyond correspondence, video conferencing, and voice mail: Masters Degree courses in nursing. *Journal of Nursing Education, 38*(6), 267-271.

Zlotolow, D.S. (2002). Case Study: San Jose State develops an online masters program in Occupational therapy. *T.H.E. Journal, 29*(11), 28-30.

Appendix A

Panel of Experts and Academic Qualification

Panel of Experts and Academic Qualifications

Marilyn Klakovich	DNSc.- University of San Diego MSN- California State University, Los Angeles MS/Healthcare Management- California State University, Los Angeles
Stephanie Vaughn	Ph.D- University of San Diego MSN- Southern Illinois University
Maria Bedroni	Ed.D., Institutional Management- Pepperdine University MN- University of California, Los Angeles
Melva Giles	Ed.D, Institutional Management- Pepperdine University MSN- California State University, Dominguez Hills
Janet Blenner	Ph.D- New York University MA, Nursing- New York University

Appendix B

Sample Email Solicitation

Dear,

I would like to thank your for your willingness to assist me in research efforts. As you already know, I am a doctoral candidate at Pepperdine University in the Graduate School of Education and Psychology. I am sending this email so that you may share information concerning this research study with your alumni. This study has been submitted for review and has been approved by the following institutional Review Boards: Pepperdine University Protocol # __E0505D03_____, University of Phoenix Protocol , and University of California at Los Angeles Protocol #__G0601-050-1__.

The purpose of my research is to explore the lived experiences of student learning in alternative Master of Science in Nursing Programs in order to gain an understanding of the meaning of this experience and its' impact on the student. For the purpose of this research, alternative refers to programs that employ methods of instruction such as online education, team learning, and/or accelerated curriculum.

The criteria for participant selection are that individual must have completed an alternative Master of Science in Nursing Program within the last three years (2002-2005). Participation in the study will take approximately two hours of the participants' time for the initial meeting and possibly an additional thirty minutes on a later date for a follow up interview.

During the initial meeting, participants will be given a complete explanation of the purpose of the study, risks, and benefits, and will be asked to sign and informed consent form. Prior to the interview, the participant will be asked to complete a demographic data questionnaire. The interview will be tape recorded. Transcripts of the interview will be prepared by a professional stenographer and will be available for review by the participant if requested.

The potential risks of participation in this study include interview fatigue and emotional distress. If for any reason that the participant becomes fatigued, he/she will be offered a break. If at any time the participant becomes uncomfortable in regards to speaking about a particular subject or event, he/she may choose not to continue that element of the discussion. Potential benefits to the individual include the opportunity to contribute to the understanding of alternative education as well as to contribute to the profession of nursing a whole.

There will be no monetary compensation provided to participants in this study, but there contribution will be much appreciated. Please share this email with your alumni and if they are interested in participating in this study have them contact me directly by phone or by email.

Thank you again for your contribution to this research effort. I look forward to hearing further from you.

Sincerely,

Mikel W. Hand EdD(c), MSN, RN, OCN, CNA, BC
XXXXXXXXXX
XXXXXXXXXXXX,
XXXXXXXXXXXXX

Appendix C

Demographic Data Questionnaire

Demographic Data   Number_____

1. Age_____

2. Ethnicity (Please Check)
    ___ African American
    ___ Asian
    ___ Caucasian
    ___ Hispanic
    ___ Native American
    ___ Other (Please specify)

3. Education   Date of Completion
    Master of Science in Nursing
    Graduate Degrees in other Fields (Specify)   _____
    Bachelor of Science in Nursing   _____
    Bachelor other field (Specify)   _____
    Other   _____
4. Family Composition
    Relationship   Age   Gender

    _____

    _____
    _____
    _____

5. Employed during the course of the program
    Yes____   No____   If Yes, Part-time or Full-time_____

    Position held during the program_____

    Number of hours worked per week during your MSN program_____

6. Which of the following best describes your MSN major?
    Nurse Practitioner_____
    Clinical Nurse Specialist_____
    Nurse Administrator _____
    Educator _____
    Other (Please Specify) _____

7. Number of courses taken at one time during the MSN program
    1 course_____

2-3 courses_____
Other (Please Specify)

8. Distance of travel to attend class

   _____

9. Frequency of face to face class meetings

   _____

Appendix D

Lead in Question and Potential Probative Questions

Lead in Question and Potential Probative Questions

Standard lead in question (used for all participants)- Tell me a story about what the experience of learning in an alternative Master of Science in Nursing was like for you.

Follow Up Probes in the Event of no Response

Experience/Behavior Probes

    a. How did you end up deciding to enroll in your program?

    b. Who were the people that you first talked to about enrolling in the program?

    c. If I had been with you on your first day of class, what might I have observed about your first day of experience?

    d. What was your first conversation with your classmates about?

Opinions/Values Probes

    e. As you reflect on your experience of graduate education, what are the things that come to your mind as most significant?

    f. What do you value the most about the experience you have had in your MSN programs?

    g. As you think back, what were the things that sustained you through the process of completing your degree?

    h. If you were given the opportunity to talk with other graduate students, what would in your opinion be the most important elements to share with them about your experience and why.

Knowledge Probes

    i. Tell me what you know about traditional programs that may have influenced your decision to choose your particular MSN program.

j. What can you tell me about that has changed in your professional knowledge base as a result of this experience?

Sensory Probe

k. Take just a few moments and reflect on your entire educational experience. Describe what comes to mind. What do you see? What do you hear? What does the experience of your program mean to you?

Standard Closing Questions (used for all participants) - Is there anything else about this experience you would like to share? Is there anything we have talked about that you would like to share further?

Appendix E

Sample Composition

Sample Composition

Participant Age	Ethnicity	Gender
21-25 = 1	Caucasion- 11	Female- 13
26-30= 0	African American- 1	Male- 1
31-35= 1	Pacific Islander -1	N= 14
36- 40= 2	Hispanic- 1	
41-45= 1	N= 14	
46-50= 4		
51- 55= 5		
N= 14		
Mean= 44.6		
SD= 9		

Degree Completion Yr	Family Composition	Age of children
2002- 3	Spouse- 10	Mean = 16. 3
2003- 1	Children- 11	SD= 7.9
2004- 6	Inlaws- 2	Range= 2-25 yrs of age
2005- 4		

Number of Hrs/Wk Worked	Position Held	Masters Specialization
10-15- 1	Staff- 6	Administrator- 8
16- 20- 1	Clinical Research- 2	Admin/Occ. Health- 1
21-25- 1	Supervisor- 1	Generalist- 3
26-30- 2	Director- 4	Educator- 2
31- 35- 0	CRNA- 1	
36- 40- 7		
> 40- 1		
Mean= 34.6		
SD= 11.4		

Number of Courses Taken at One time	Distance of Travel	Frequency of Class Meetings
Range- 1-4	Range- 0-110 miles	Range- 0-4x per term
Mean- 2.3	Mean- 27.8	Mean- 1.5 x per term
SD- 1.2	SD- 36.7	SD- 1.3

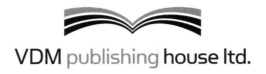

VDM publishing house ltd.

Scientific Publishing House

offers

free of charge publication

of current academic research papers, Bachelor´s Theses, Master's Theses, Dissertations or Scientific Monographs

If you have written a thesis which satisfies high content as well as formal demands, and you are interested in a remune- rated publication of your work, please send an e-mail with some initial information about yourself and your work to *info@vdm-publishing-house.com*.

Our editorial office will get in touch with you shortly.

VDM Publishing House Ltd.
Meldrum Court 17.
Beau Bassin
Mauritius
www.vdm-publishing-house.com

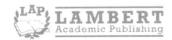
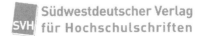

Printed in Great Britain
by Amazon.co.uk, Ltd.,
Marston Gate.